The Ultimate Vegan and Intermittent Fasting Guide:

Everything you need to lose weight healthily

by

Aidan Curtis

Copyright © 2022 by Aidan Curtis

All rights reserved.

No part of this book may be reproduced, or used in any manner without written permission of the copyright owner except for the use of quotations in a book review.

Table of Contents

INTRODUCTION 1
    THE PROBLEM WITH MAINSTREAM DIETS 8
    HEALTH & WEIGHT LOSS 13

CHAPTER 01. HISTORY OF FASTING 16
    IS FASTING STARVATION? 22

CHAPTER 02. HISTORY OF THE VEGAN DIET 26

CHAPTER 03. THE RELATIONSHIP BETWEEN IF AND HUNGER 29
    GHRELIN – THE "HUNGER" HORMONE 32
    LEPTIN – THE "SATIETY" HORMONE 34
    INSULIN – THE "ENERGY" HORMONE 36
    HOW FASTING MAKES YOU LESS HUNGRY 38

CHAPTER 04. VEGAN GUIDELINES 45
    THE CONCEPT OF VEGANISM 46
    WHAT CAN I AND CANNOT EAT? 47
    IS VEGANISM HEALTHY, AND WILL I AUTOMATICALLY LOSE WEIGHT? 51

CHAPTER 05. INTERMITTENT FASTING GUIDELINES 55

TEMPORARY SOLUTION VERSUS A LIFESTYLE CHANGE .. 56
INTERMITTENT FASTING SCHEDULE 58
HOW TO START FASTING 60
ONE-WEEK INTERMITTENT FASTING SAMPLE................. 65

CHAPTER 06. BENEFITS OF INTERMITTENT FASTING & VEGAN DIET... 66

THE PERFECT WEIGHT LOSS COMBO............................... 66
HIGHER FIBRE CONSUMPTION 72
FASTER METABOLISM FOR MORE WEIGHT LOSS................ 73
A VEGAN DIET IS MORE NUTRIENT-DENSE THAN OTHER OPTIONS... 76
A VEGAN DIET WILL LOWER YOUR BLOOD SUGAR LEVELS. 77
FASTING AND VEGANISM – RELATIONSHIP WITH FOOD .. 79
LOWER BLOOD SUGAR AND INSULIN LEVELS 84
SHARPENING YOUR SENSES WITH FASTING 85

CHAPTER 07. SIDE EFFECTS OF FASTING 94

KETO DIET? NO! KETO FLU? YES! 94
YOU MIGHT GET CONSTIPATED. 97
ELECTROLYTES IMBALANCE... 98
VARIATION IN ENERGY LEVELS.. 99

CHAPTER 08. THE WEIGHT LOSS TIPS THAT MADE ME LOSE FOUR STONES................................. 101

"COFFEE CAN TRULY BECOME AN ALLY"......................... 101

STAY AWAY FROM THE "HEALTHY PROCESSED" FOOD OPTIONS..102
TRICK YOUR BRAIN INTO THINKING YOU ARE NOT ON A DIET 103
COOKING YOUR MEALS WILL ALWAYS BE THE BEST OPTION. 104
CHANGE YOUR SNACKING HABITS. 105
DON'T ALLOW FOOD TO DOMINATE YOUR LIFE. 106
MOVE, EVEN IF AT HOME. 107
THE SHORTENED GUIDE YOU MIGHT NEED… 107

REFERENCES 112

Introduction

If you're reading this book, the chances are that just like me, you have tried countless diets throughout your life. The existing diet culture is undeniable, and it's intense. Just a few minutes watching T.V. or scrolling through social media are enough for you to see videos upon videos of people giving dieting advice, whether it be about a new food item that you can't eat if you want to burn fat or a food item that you should eat if you want to burn more fat, dieting has become a culture.

I'm aware, however, that we can't put all of the blame on "dieting culture". Most of the time, we are not happy with our bodies or with ourselves. Regardless if this concern comes from a place of worry about your physical appearance or because you're worried about your health, both are equally valid, and it's not my place to tell you that wanting to lose weight because you want to feel confident and happy with yourself is not as important as a health concern.

Regardless of why you want to lose, it's much more important to discuss the reasons you have weight management problems to begin with. We're not born overweight and obese. Instead, we develop unhealthy eating habits throughout our lives that can make us build a destructive relationship with food. The reason for that can vary, and each individual has their own history and journey with their body. However, it's important that we dive into these reasons and triggers that might have gotten you to your current place in order to take a step in the right direction in your health journey.

One of the reasons why the U.S. is currently in one of the biggest obesity crises in history is that people are often told to follow outdated advice. Although we must recognize that official institutions such as the WHO – World Health Organization have tried to lead the population towards a healthier path, we must also acknowledge that scientific information can sometimes be easily manipulated. Once you gain interest in health and nutrition and start to research more about the topic, you quickly realize that most of the things we are told are not genuinely based on strong scientific research, but instead, on older studies that were often conducted without following any of the strict guidelines that a paper must follow today.

I'm not really saying all of the information that you have heard is incorrect. A lot of the dieting advice might actually be helpful. However, there are some central beliefs when it comes to health and weight loss that can actually do more harm than good to your health. Because we place so much trust in official institutions' guidelines about eating, many people actually try to follow the same old "eat less, and work out more" advice. But is it this easy? If so, how come millions of people are becoming obese every year, with the numbers growing even more every year? Is it the people's fault? Is it my fault? Maybe was it your own fault?

For many people, obesity is often linked to a lack of discipline. Society sees obese individuals as people who simply fail to take control of their lives and how they eat. People who lost control over their own health. They aren't very friendly with us, and obese individuals often have to deal with strangers' judgment on top of their own feelings about themselves and their bodies. It's important to mention that obesity is officially considered a chronic disease by WHO. Although we can't completely ignore the fact that most of the time, we consciously make bad eating choices, we can also recognize that the disease is multifaceted. Hormones will play a part in it. Other diseases can also make you gain weight. The medication that you take can also have weight gain as a side effect, and so on. So, it is important to take these other factors into consideration as well.

Now, we have already considered two different factors: Outdated research and the multifaceted nature of obesity, but there is more. Aside from these two factors, we must also recognize that obesity is, sometimes, a consequence of an eating disorder, or at the very least, a result of disordered eating behaviours. The main difference between the two is that while eating disorders are mental illnesses with many symptoms, disordered eating behaviour is one symptom that can represent, or not, an eating disorder.

For example, anorexia nervosa and bulimia are both eating disorders. On the other hand, binge eating is often considered a disordered eating behaviour because even people who don't have an eating disorder can sometimes have binge eating episodes. Don't think so? Think about your latest Thanksgiving dinner. Better yet, think about your last Christmas meal with your family. How much did you eat? Did you feel good after it? Felt like you could run a marathon? Yes? Well, the answer is probably the complete opposite. You most likely ate enough to the point of feeling sick and being unable to move for several minutes after the meal. Does this mean that you have an eating disorder? Not necessarily, although medical advice can help in this situation. However, at the very least, this showcases that you do, indeed, have disordered eating behaviours. Although this might be shocking to hear, eating to the point of feeling abdominal pain and experiencing what is called a "food coma", when you are unable to move and do anything after a meal, isn't "normal". It's anything but healthy as well.

People develop disordered eating behaviours for a series of reasons. However, emotional eating is one of the most common factors. Do you know that huge craving you get in the middle of your workday and how you literally cannot wait to get home and eat? This is a clear example of emotional eating. More often than not, we have these cravings after a long day of work, when we're stressed and tired. During moments like these, all we want to do is eat the first sugary food we can find. This happens because food becomes a source of relief and pleasure. Maybe even the only source of comfort available. While some people might decide to relax by drinking a glass of wine or smoking, for example, some people run to food.

Emotional eating can also be a consequence of chemical reactions in the brain. Here, we are essentially talking about food addiction, and there is a reason for that. Sugar is highly addictive, and most of the processed foods that we buy at the supermarket are packed with it. In our bodies, sugar activates neurotransmitters related to the pleasure sensors in our brain. When done repeatedly, this can become an addiction, in a way that whenever you feel like you need a dose of relief and pleasure, you will seek sugary food sources.

To better understand this, think about the times when you needed to take medicine, for example. When you have easy access to pills, and you have headaches, for example, you will take the medication in order to stop the pain. Over-the-counter remedies offer a temporary solution to the pain, but they fail to eliminate the actual source of the pain. If you are suffering from constant headaches, then you will take multiple pills throughout many different days. With time, your body becomes used to the effects of the medication, and they stop working as well as before. Now, you need to take even more pills in order to get rid of your headaches, creating dependency. Taking more pills only feeds the cycle.

The same happens with food. Once you realize that eating your favourite cookie brings you an immediate sense of pleasure, you start to constantly eat them whenever you feel the slightest amount of stress. It becomes a habit, but eventually, eating only one cookie won't make you feel as good as before. Being so, you eat more cookies. This time, maybe you will eat a bowl of pasta too. This only makes you more dependent on the sugar to feel better about yourself, when a much more effective approach would be to try to understand why you're running to food, to begin with. This goal, however, can't be achieved by following a mainstream diet.

The Problem with Mainstream Diets

Now we know that the reason you might be failing your weight loss goals is that weight gain can have multiple different reasons. Being so, one simple solution will hardly fix all of the issues that might be making you choose food to feel better about yourself. Nonetheless, this sheds light on why so many of us keep trying mainstream diets. When nothing seems to work, and the official guidelines do nothing for us, our only choice becomes to keep trying popular diets until one of them works.

Then, another cycle begins. See if this sounds familiar to you. Every week, you promise yourself that you'll start a new diet by Monday. Maybe this was triggered by some news that you saw about a new popular diet that has gained the headlines. Perhaps you saw a video on social media that may have led to the decision to try something new. You research everything about the diet. Maybe you even buy new workout clothes. You prepare yourself for what you believe might be your very last diet because this time, it will work. You go to the grocery store and buy all of the food items that are allowed under the new guidelines that you're about to follow. You also remove junk food from your kitchen to avoid temptation. Everything is ready.

By Monday, you start. You begin cooking your own meals at home. You feel good and determined that this time you will get all of the results that you want. For the first day, maybe, things go well, and you believe that this might be it. By the second day, things already don't feel the same. You crave that sugary coffee and wonder if you could maybe still buy it even though you're on a diet. The day doesn't go well.

By the next day, you're tired. You don't want to keep thinking about what to eat anymore, and you just want to have food freedom. The Guidelines that seemed to excite you now sound like torture, and you convince yourself that it will be impossible to keep following them for an extended period of time – which would be necessary for you to get the results that you want. Thus, your brain convinces you that the only possible solution is to give up altogether. What's the point of wasting time today only to give up tomorrow anyway?

Whether you gave up because you were going through sugar withdrawal symptoms, or maybe your disordered eating behaviours took the best of you, or perhaps even your emotional attachment to food – an issue that is still very much unresolved – something prevented you from succeeding. Regardless, this cycle ended, but you won't give up, will you? After two days without following any specific diet, you start yet again thinking that you should lose weight. Maybe it was a video on social media. Perhaps you saw a headline about a new diet. Maybe…

… The mainstream diet is to blame…

Mainstream diets are often crafted with the goal of being marketable. Dieting is an industry. When a new diet becomes popular, so will the products and services surrounding the diet guidelines. This means profit for the businesses offering these products. In this case, trust me. They don't really want you to lose weight permanently. After all, if you do, then you don't need to buy these products and services anymore, right?

The Gluten-Free Diet is the perfect example of what I'm explaining. A few years ago, many celebrities started to promote a Gluten-free way of eating to their audiences. This not only led to many people following the diet, but countless "No-Gluten" products began to appear on grocery stores all around the country magically. However, Gluten is a protein, one of the three macronutrients found in most of the foods that we eat. For most of us, the protein is completely harmless, and the only people who should actively avoid any gluten food source are those with celiac disease. This disease makes the body unable to digest Gluten, causing damage to the digestive tract. If you don't have it, then there is no active need to remove Gluten from your diet altogether.

This highlights a common problem with most mainstream diets. Their guidelines simply do not have any actual scientific logic behind them. You can very well eat a Gluten-free diet and still gain weight because Gluten isn't directly associated with weight gain, for most people, to begin with. Diets that encourage you only to eat protein, or only drink juices for a week, or maybe eat a soup for every meal will often fail to provide basic reasoning as to why you should do so.

By following these diets and achieving no results, you start to resent food as if it was something terrible, which makes you gain weight. The problem here is in the diet, not in the food. Most of these diets are focused on one thing and one thing only, which is weight loss. Thus, they are all essentially the same diet written in different words. A soup diet or juice diet has as its primary purpose to reduce the number of calories you're eating, for example, but only lead you to failure because there is a lot more to trying to lose weight than simply eating less.

Diets like these lead to the creation of products that will often be marketed as "healthy" even when they aren't. Most of them don't forbid the consumption of these products but rather encourage it. For example, Low Sodium, Low Sugar, Low Gluten, Low Lactose, etc. products are often, just as their names suggest, Low on something specifically. Does this mean they are healthy? Far from that. Processed "diet" products are still loaded with preservatives, food dyes, and other additives. Not to mention, these products are, deep down, made for people with specific needs.

Just like it happens with gluten-free products, low sugar products are often the best choice for people who have diabetes. On the other hand, the same products will have alarming amounts of sodium or fat in order to preserve the taste and texture that is appealing to consumers. The same happens with other products. Low Sodium products are merely low sodium, which means they can still contain alarming amounts of sugar and fats. Processed "dieting products", although labelled as such, are most of the time not weight loss friendly. That's why you must know the difference between a diet for weight loss and a diet for better health and a consequential weight loss.

Health & Weight Loss

Most of the mainstream diets were never designed with the goal of improving your health but instead as an attempt to cause quick weight loss. Highly restrictive diets are good examples of this. Most of them have very defined guidelines that either don't have any reasoning or are purely based on principles that would put your body under a lot of stress to force a quick weight loss. I want to make it clear that it is possible to lose weight in an unhealthy way. It is possible to force your body into losing a lot of water weight, for example. It is possible to drastically restrict your calories in order to put you in a massive calorie deficit. Would this be beneficial for your health? Most likely not, mainly because your body needs energy in order to function. However, it can lead to quick weight loss nonetheless.

Keep in mind that if your diet is temporary, so will your weight loss. Most people have the intention of starting a diet in order to lose weight but only do it temporarily. Then, they spend a few weeks or months following the guidelines while seeing results but are often eager to go back to their usual ways of eating. Listen, your normal way of eating is what made you gain weight, to begin with. Changing your habits in order to lose weight and then changing it back to how you used to eat before will only make you gain weight again, causing the yoyo effect.

This cycle of losing a bit of weight and then gaining it double the amount back is hugely damaging to both your physical and mental health and should be avoided. Being so, the best approach when it comes to deciding which strategy you'll follow is by paying attention to two factors: Did these guidelines survive the test of time, and are these guidelines scientifically proven? In this book, I'm sharing the two strategies that, when combined, made me lose four stones and, most importantly, allowed me to maintain my low weight instead of gaining it all back. The information you'll read in the following chapters is backed up by scientific research throughout the decades. By the end of this project, you'll have all the information and tools needed in order to implement them into your routine today. I'm talking about Intermittent Fasting and the Vegan Diet. Throughout this book, you'll notice how these two strategies complement each other, creating the most perfect weight loss and health combo. Welcome!

Chapter 01. History of Fasting

When we talk about diet and strategies to lose weight, there is a common theme: "What we can and cannot eat", besides of course, how much we can eat. Diets are geared towards what we eat, food combinations, and macronutrients, but this is not the case with Intermittent Fasting. The only thing that matters to practitioners of Fasting is "when" you eat, nothing more.

Despite having gained popularity in recent years, Fasting is an ancient practice, almost a tradition. However, it was not used for weight loss but for its other benefits such as improved concentration, prevention of ageing, etc. Humans fasted, at first, for lack of choice. In the past, there were no supermarkets and delivery services that could bring your meal to your doorsteps in just a few minutes. Instead, humans needed to hunt and plant their food, which means that they weren't always available. Being so, humans ate freely when food was available but would spend more prolonged periods of time fasting when they couldn't find food. However, even while our civilizations evolved, Fasting was never truly left behind.

All around the world, Fasting became a tradition in many different cultures. Philosophers recommended it as a treatment option for many diseases and a general method to enhance health. Hippocrates, considered the father of medicine by many, is one of the biggest names in history to recommend Fasting. He emphasized that "To eat when you are sick is to feed your illness". In addition to him, Plutarch also suggested patients to practice Fasting in order to heal instead of taking medication by writing, "Instead of using medicine, better fast today".

Researchers of Intermittent Fasting also highlighted that the practice seemed natural and easily observed in nature. They were referring to the fact that most animals, when sick, will willingly fast while they recover. Initially, this idea can sound puzzling. After all, don't we need to eat in order to become strong and healthier? Then why would animals in the wild make the decision not to eat when they are injured? The reason for this instinct is believed to be protection. One of the most significant benefits of Fasting (which we will discuss later) is the enhancement of cognitive skills. This means that you feel more attentive and alert during the Fast, necessary skills for weakened animals. Therefore, it is believed that the instinct to stop eating when injured allows them to become more aware of the dangers while they recover. After all, it is known that the period of greatest vulnerability for many animals is right after a large meal.

However, they are not the only ones. This happens with humans too. You can probably recall many different times throughout your life when you overate. Thanksgiving and Christmas dinners are often good examples. Maybe you skipped a meal by accident and decided to compensate on the next meal as well. Regardless of what made you overeat during a meal; The truth is that right after, you will feel lethargic and sleepy. There is even an official name for this phenomenon, "Food Coma". Food Coma happens right after you overate to the point of discomfort. Running, reading, and solving problems will probably sound like torture once you finished your meal. The same happens with animals. If they are injured, they are already slower and weak, so eating would only make them more vulnerable.

Food Coma can also be explained by looking at how our bodies digest food. When you have a big meal, your body will need to use a lot of energy to digest and absorb the nutrients. This is the first reason why you become so lethargic. Second, most of the blood and oxygen in your body will be directed to your digestive system to aid the digestive process. This leaves your brain with less blood and oxygen, which explains why reading a book or solving a math problem can sound almost impossible after a huge meal. When we understand this, it becomes easier to see what Hippocrates meant when he said, "To eat when you are sick is to feed the illness".

You see, knowing how much energy and effort your body spends trying to digest food, it becomes clear that eating all of the time can quickly become a problem. Suppose you have the habit of having a meal every three hours, for example. In that case, this cycle of redirecting all of your body's energy and resources to your digestive system keeps happening throughout the day. It's almost as if by doing this, you never allow your body to focus on other things, such as eliminating waste and detoxing itself. Once people realized that Fasting allowed the body to heal from many diseases naturally, the practice gained even more popularity.

Philip Paracelsus, the leading name when it comes to toxicology, additionally had even more grounded convictions when it came to Fasting. He said that "Fasting is the greatest remedy", and even Benjamin Franklin, an enormous name in American history, additionally wrote that "The best of all medicines is resting and fasting". Although the majority of the names mentioned strongly advocated for Fasting as a type of treatment for illnesses, as it allowed the body to recuperate without the "workload" of processing food, we should also remember that Fasting has spiritual implications.

Indeed, quick research will show the connections between Fasting and essentially every single religion in the world. Supporters will use the method both as a type of selflessness act or as a tool for spiritual development. Religious "Leaders" such as Buddha, Jesus Christ, and Muhammed urged their devotees to practice Fasting when looking for answers for their difficulties or when needing to better connect with their divine beings. The final goal was to purge the souls, attempting to cleanse the spirit in order to allow a more profound relationship with their religions and their leaders. Fasting is likewise traced back as part of the culture of innumerable societies, as it was referred to as being advantageous for both the body and psyche. When we move forward a few years, the practice kept growing in popularity and gathering even more supporters past the religious beliefs.

In addition to philosophers and historians, modern medicine also reinforces the importance of Fasting. Dr Ancel Keys, pioneer of one of the most famous diets, the Mediterranean diet, was inspired by the people of Crete, located in Greece, to create the diet for their enviable health. However, Dr Ancel Keys ignored another method used by almost the entire population of the island, Fasting, which is mainly responsible for the health of the local population. Unfortunately, Fasting was still completely left out in his adaptation of the Mediterranean eating regimen. In any case, being seemingly perhaps the most all-around established practice ever, Fasting has become almost a "secret" and yet effective tool to health improvement and weight loss, and you currently have the chance to use it for your benefit.

Is fasting starvation?

Before we jump into the following chapters about Fasting and the Vegan Diet, we should comprehend the idea of fasting in itself and how this eating pattern became popular. And Yes, Fasting is an eating pattern, not an eating regimen or a diet. For this reason, it's not about changing what you eat, but rather when you eat, which will provide all of the benefits associated with the practice. In any case, one of the essential points of discussion about whether one should fast or not be about whether one is starving themselves while fasting.

Intermittent Fasting is a food strategy where there is a **voluntary** absence of food for a certain period of time. This definition is essential, as many people believe that Fasting means hunger, and this is not true. Starvation occurs and can be defined as moments when there is an involuntary absence of food. A Homeless person who unfortunately doesn't have enough money to buy any food is starving. Deciding to skip breakfast and only eating lunch is fasting. Think of Fasting as being controlled and planned for health, weight loss, and even for spiritual reasons. After all, Fasting is a common practice in most religions for the purpose of purifying the body, but never as a form of starvation. This can be further explained when we take a look at when Fasting was used in "modern" medicine.

Around 500 B.C., in the Hippocratic era, patients with epilepsy were subjected to a treatment that involved prolonged Fasting to control seizures. In this fast, only water intake was allowed in order to maintain hydration. Although it was not feasible to keep the patients fasting, there are reports that epileptic seizures were significantly reduced. Then, in 1911, two Parisian doctors - Guelpa and Marie - developed a study on the treatment of epilepsy with prolonged Fasting, subjecting 20 children and adults to this strategy and reported that, during treatment, the crises were less intense. At the end of the First World War, the American physical educator Bernarr Macfadden published in the magazine "Physical Culture", an article that reported the benefit of fasting from three days to three weeks in the treatment and prognosis of some diseases, including epilepsy.

From then on, Fasting remained as a treatment option for those with epilepsy. Along with the Keto diet, Greek doctors would prescribe the practice to treat not only epilepsy but also numerous other medical issues. Hippocrates, which, as you know, was a great supporter of the method, further supported the utilization of Fasting as an epilepsy treatment until the practice did become a standard tool and resource for treating and preventing seizures well as other conditions.

When other treatment options were starting to be developed, Fasting and even the Keto Diet were kind of left behind. However, they were quickly reintroduced as a treatment method when the results obtained with other treatments weren't as good. Thus, fasting kept being used, especially to help children with epilepsy, as an attempt to reduce their seizures.

The reason why it is so important to take a look at fasting history is so that we can highlight that, in one way or the other, Fasting was always associated with health in the first place. It wasn't a strategy created with the goal of merely weight loss, and being so the practice can bring countless benefits to your health that are beyond a smaller number on the scale. Instead, the practice only began to gain popularity in the "dieting world" when new studies about the method started to come back with alarming results regarding weight loss. As more studies were made, we slowly started to understand the mechanisms that made intermittent fasting an excellent tool for weight loss as well. Today, you can implement Fasting to your routine regardless if you want to lose weight or not, as it can also benefit your health. We'll discuss the mechanisms of Intermittent Fasting in the following few chapters.

Chapter 02. History of the Vegan Diet

Siddhartha Gautama, also known as Buddha, was one of the first names in history to talk with his followers about the importance of an animal-free diet. Along with him, Pythagoras also encouraged humans to stop consuming animal protein. His reasons, however, were primarily ethical. Nonetheless, Buddha and Siddhartha became the first references of a conscience that would later help to shape Veganism as we know it today. However, at the time, Veganism was only giving its first few baby steps.

Moving forward many years later, in the first century, the Greek philosopher Plutarch wrote many times about stopping eating animal protein as well, which further pushed for the practice to become a viable option for many people. Still, only in the 15th century onwards was there substantial growth in the number of people and celebrities who openly talked about Vegetarianism as more of a "philosophy of life", not only for ethical reasons but also because of health concerns about what animal protein might do to our bodies.

The official term that we use today is "veganism", which was coined in 1944 by a group of "six non-dairy vegetarians", summoned to a meeting by Englishman Donald Watson. During a meeting in Birmingham, United Kingdom, they started to ponder what term could define their eating habits and lifestyles. Their decision was then for the word "vegan", which was created from the combination of the first three with the last two letters of the word "**VEG**etari**AN**". In that very same year, the first-ever "Vegan Society" was created. The very first official definition of the term would only be defined in 1979 when the term was deemed a

"[...] A philosophy and way of life that seeks to exclude - as far as possible and practicable - all forms of exploitation, and cruelty, from animals to food, clothing or any other purpose; and, by extension, it promotes the development and use of animal-free alternatives for the benefit of humans, animals and the environment. In food terms, it denotes the practice of rejecting all products

derived wholly or partially from animals". Source: PetaIndia

For example, the official World Vegan Day, which happens on November 1st, is thanks to the institution's anniversary date. This is vital for you to know because the Vegan Society will grant certification for vegan products to be labelled as such, being responsible for more than 22,000 products and services worldwide. Although the history of the Vegan diet is brief, today, the diet is one of the most popular diet options used for both weight loss purposes, health, and also ethical and moral reasons. To me, however, the diet was essential for my weight loss journey success, and I'm happy to tell you how I did it.

Chapter 03. The relationship between IF and Hunger

You already know that Fasting and starvation are entirely different things and that you shouldn't use both of the terms as if they meant the same thing. However, even while knowing that you're not starving yourself while fasting, you might still fear hunger. If you go long hours without eating, the obvious consequence is that you will feel hunger, correct? The fear of having an increase in their appetite is something that makes individuals avoid fasting altogether. Little do they know that the results will be ultimately the opposite, but one step at a time. This belief that you will feel extreme hunger while Fasting is a consequence of one of our primary dieting advice. The idea that you must eat every three hours to keep your digestion running and allow for weight loss. Other people might simply believe that they can't go long hours without eating because they are used to always having a snack by their sides, the habit of constantly chewing something throughout the day. We also have "official meal times". Thus, during breakfast, lunch, and dinner, we are expected to eat, even if we're not hungry.

To understand why Fasting will actually reduce your hunger instead of increasing it, we must learn about three hormones: Insulin, Ghrelin, and Leptin, the ones directly related to our hunger cues and energy. Can you remember some of those days when you began salivating when you returned home and your friends or roommates were cooking? Why do you think you feel the need to always buy popcorn at the movies once you smell it? How many times did you daydream about that piece of cake that you left on your fridge, hoping that no one would eat while you were outside of the house?

Allow me to tell you the truth: In all of these situations, the chances that you were actually hungry are minimal. Instead, this is simply a result of cravings. This is essentially wanting to eat, regardless of being hungry or merely craving to chew something while watching the movie. Knowing how to recognize when you are actually hungry and without energy – You'll learn that hunger is mainly connected with energy rather than food - from when you are merely bored and want to chew something or when you buy food purely out of habit will be essential during Intermittent Fasting, and this process has a lot to do with the three hormones that I mentioned.

I'm talking about something called hormonal regulation, the one thing that will control all of your hunger cues, your satiety and will essentially tell your body when to eat and when to stop eating. All of these actions are controlled by these three hormones, and when they become imbalanced due to a vast number of reasons, your entire hunger system changes. Essentially, your body can tell you to eat more even when you shouldn't, and trying to fight against this urge becomes almost impossible. One of the primary reasons why Intermittent Fasting is so powerful for weight loss is precisely because it offers hormone regulation as one of its primary benefits, meaning that while fasting, all of these hormones will be working correctly, telling you to eat only when you are actually in need of energy. This is how they work:

Ghrelin – The "Hunger" Hormone

The number one function of the hunger hormone, as the name suggests, is to send signals to the brain to tell you that it is time to eat. Being so, whenever you feel the need to eat something, it is because Ghrelin levels are high. It's worth mentioning that dieting, for example, is known for increasing Ghrelin levels. After all, in most diets with calorie restrictions, you're not actually following the correct "protocol" to provide your body with energy while still losing weight. Being so scared of running out of fuel, your body increases Ghrelin levels, and your appetite becomes uncontrollable.

Naturally, Ghrelin usually is very effective at warning the body when to eat, yet as you may imagine, when these hormone levels are all over the place, you may experience the side effects, which consist of constant hunger regardless of how much you eat. You must comprehend that your appetite has more to do with your energy levels than how much food you are consuming. You might believe they are the same thing, as food is, after all, energy in the form of calories. However, the main difference here lies in how the body uses this energy. You'll see more about this when learning about Insulin. However, one good example of how this process works is by thinking that the vast majority of us don't feel hungry when we wake up and at the beginning of the day. Initially, this might sound weird, as when you wake up, you have gone through at least six or eight hours without eating. Being so, how come we can feel less hungry in the morning, judging by the Ghrelin levels, after spending so many hours without eating?

Your gut is responsible for producing the hormone Ghrelin, which is likewise called lenomorelin. When your energy levels drop, the hormone is released and travels to your hypothalamus, the part of your brain related to hunger. There, it will activate hunger cues, and your appetite will increase. As your body and brain like comfort and always choose the easiest way of doing things, you will most likely end up craving sugary foods because they contain the most significant calories per gram. Your appetite levels will be directly related to your Ghrelin levels, which means that extremely high hormone levels equal extreme hunger, and being so, keeping

Ghrelin levels on the lower side is the best option when trying to lose weight, for example.

… And how can these hormone levels become imbalanced then?

Obesity is one of the reasons, and studies show that when you have a higher BMI – Body Mass Index, especially in the obese category, you have higher Ghrelin levels when compared to people who are considered to have a "normal" weight. Hence, trying to lose in itself is perhaps the most ideal approach to control ghrelin levels. You might wonder then how this would be possible. If obesity can lead to higher Ghrelin levels and higher Ghrelin levels can lead to obesity, then how can you break the cycle? You will soon discover that Fasting is perhaps the best method for reducing ghrelin levels and try to achieve hormonal balance to break free from the cycle. For now, understanding that this hormone is related to energy and hunger is enough.

Leptin – The "Satiety" Hormone

Being essentially the polar opposite of Ghrelin, Leptin, or "satiety hormone", is mainly produced in the fat cells. As the name suggests, its function is to tell your body to stop eating or reduce your appetite, which implies that it is a hunger suppressant. Through a series of different mechanisms, Leptin will basically hinder Ghrelin, reducing its levels in the body. Initially, when leptin levels are on the higher side, it blocks the production and release of Ghrelin. With the second mechanism, Leptin also blocks the Ghrelin receptors, which will stop the connection between hormone and receptor from happening. Being so, Ghrelin becomes unable to increase your appetite.

Likewise, Leptin increases thermogenesis, which further supports weight loss. Have you at any point come across an article about a specific type of food called "thermogenic"? The term refers to food items that, while being digested, require more energy from the body. During the digestive process, the body will produce more warmth, which pushes for more fat burning. Thermogenic food items will also boost Metabolism, which is not only great for your energy levels but can also make you burn more calories throughout the day. Accordingly, keeping up higher leptin levels is fundamental for any weight loss strategy.

Insulin – The "Energy" Hormone

This hormone produced by the pancreas has the capacity of moving glucose from your circulatory system to the cells, where they will be used as a source of energy. When you eat a meal that contains a lot of sugar food sources, your body will break the sugar down into glucose. The glucose will sit in your bloodstream, which makes the body signal the release of Insulin. The hormone will then try to remove the glucose from the blood and store it in the cells. The bigger your meal is, the more Insulin is needed in order to keep your blood sugar levels low. This means that a high amount of sugar will equal what we call an Insulin spike.

Thinking about this concept, you probably know that when you take too much medication, it will eventually lose its power, and you will need to take even more pills in order to notice the effect, right? The same happens here. If you are eating back-to-back meals containing a lot of sugar, then your insulin levels will remain high. The same principle from the pills will apply here. When this happens constantly, your body will stop responding to the hormone, and your body will produce even more in order to try and maintain your glucose levels down, which just further harms the cycle. When this happens, you officially develop what is called "Insulin Resistance", which can prevent you from losing weight and become dangerous to your health. These are some of the symptoms:

- Lower energy levels
- Food Coma, when you overeat to the point of feeling abdominal pain.
- Cravings, especially for sugary foods.
- Difficulty maintaining your focus and ability to concentrate.
- Weight gain and increase in fat percentage.
- Lower HDL, the good cholesterol that can enhance heart health.
- Difficulty losing weight despite dieting.

Remember that appetite is mainly connected with cell energy levels than food in itself. On the off chance that your body is unable to respond to Insulin appropriately, then energy will fail to reach the cells regardless of how much you eat. Being so, it is entirely possible to overeat and still starve the cells simply because of Insulin Resistance. When your cells are starved, your body will keep sending signals for you to eat because your energy levels are dropping. But as you know, eating won't fix the issue since the main problem is hormonal. Then how do we fix this? By following a method of eating that can promote Insulin regulation: Fasting.

How Fasting makes you less hungry

Now you know how all three of these hormones work. Being so, we can start to understand how they will function during the Fasting, especially when it comes to controlling and reducing appetite. For example, in one study[1], patients were submitted to a 33 hour fast. Throughout the entire study, every 20 minutes, their Ghrelin levels were measured. This single study brings up a lot of points of discussion for our thesis that Fasting can make you less hungry. Initially, as I have mentioned, Ghrelin levels are the lowest as soon as we wake up. This piece of information already changes everything you might know about weight loss and hunger, as people usually think we need to eat in order to not be hungry. This study shows that it isn't this easy, and this statement is simply not true. How come you feel less hungry after spending a good six or eight hours without eating? Shouldn't your Ghrelin levels be the highest in the morning then? This discloses that appetite and food are not as related as we might suspect they are. Eating doesn't really make you less hungry, and following the same principle, not eating (Fasting) doesn't make you hungrier either.

This study likewise showed that Ghrelin levels are typically high during regular meal times, like breakfast, lunch, and dinner, for example. If you have your snacking time in the same hour every day, you might also experience higher Ghrelin levels during these times as well. This implies that you can make dietary patterns that will impact your appetite —eating becomes a habit, instead of something that you do when you arc hungry, as your body becomes used to receiving food at these specific times. This explains why Ghrelin levels are higher during these times of the day, and they will also increase during your usual snack times, even if you ate before, for example.

The central issue here is that the study additionally showed that Ghrelin levels would increase during these times, yes. However, they would go back to normal after a couple of hours. Remember that patients in this study were fasting, so they did not eat. Being so, this study became great scientific proof that hunger **comes in waves**. As your ghrelin levels increase during mealtime, you become hungry. However, even if you fast, your Ghrelin levels will decrease regardless. You probably experienced this many times throughout your life as well.

Consider a day when you were genuinely busy and didn't have the opportunity to eat. When it was time for your meal, you most likely felt hunger and a longing to eat thanks to the high Ghrelin levels. However, let's suppose that you are too busy at the moment and you simply ignore it. After a few hours, you suddenly realized you weren't even hungry anymore, even though you felt like you really wanted to eat before. This is an excellent way to illustrate how Ghrelin and Leptin work and how they will impact your appetite in case you don't eat. The desire to eat will come in weaves, meaning it will go away regardless if you eat or not.

Okay, but does this mean the hormone levels won't continually increase throughout the day? Yes. The study showed that towards the end of the process, after they completed a full day of Fasting, when Ghrelin levels were measured, they had stayed stable during the entire day, even though participants were still fasting. This implies that not eating for over 24 hours didn't increase the overall Ghrelin levels at all. Notwithstanding the fact that they ate or not, their "appetite" levels remained the same. Ultimately, their final hormone levels graph measured towards the end of the study showed that after all 33 hours of Fasting, the participant's Ghrelin levels were still around the same as before they began the fast. Putting it simply, by following a 33-hour fast, when looking exclusively at the Ghrelin levels, participants were no hungrier than they were before they had begun the study. Different papers further demonstrated the same results. In another study[2], participants had their Ghrelin levels measured while following an 84-hour fast. At the end of the study, the results showed that participants' Ghrelin levels were actually lower after 84 hours of the fast. Thus, it's fair to say that people were actually less hungry after fasting for 84 hours than they were before they started the fast. Again, when looking exclusively at Ghrelin levels.

Papers like the two listed are extraordinary evidence that not only ends the discussion of whether Fasting makes you hungrier but also reinforces that the practice will do the exact opposite, reducing your appetite, which can, of course, support weight loss. Knowing this is vital because it shows that you can actually follow an intermittent fasting cycle without worrying about "slowing down your metabolism" or "starving" because you know that if you do it correctly, you will also feel better mentally and physically while also feeling less hunger. All of this will further help you during your weight loss journey.

Aside from Fasting, your diet will deeply impact how your hormone levels behave as well, and when Ghrelin and Leptin levels are imbalanced, changing your diet and becoming healthier becomes almost like fighting against what your brain is telling your body to do. No matter how disciplined and determined you are, this is a difficult task.

A better approach is to work towards balancing the hormone levels and make your body help you lose weight instead of going against it. Keep in mind that imbalanced hormone levels will boost your cravings, increase your appetite levels, and damage your energy production.

At the point when we understand how the hormones work in our bodies, we discover that weight loss isn't simply a question of willpower, which is what society will often tell us. Being so, to lose weight successfully, you must first try to fix what might be causing the weight gain in the first place, whether it be hormonal issues, emotional eating, disordered eating behaviours, and more. Why bother battling your body when you can make some changes to make your body work towards weight loss instead? Although you probably tried many diets throughout your life, and would always make sure that you were eating every three hours, which made you not understand what you were doing wrong, now you know, no diet will work unless you try to fix the root of the problem. With Fasting, you have the opportunity to work on all of them. Stick around for the Intermittent Fasting Guidelines in the following chapters.

Chapter 04. Vegan Guidelines

The Vegan Diet has been popular for a long time, but you could probably notice a sudden increase in said popularity in the past three years, which made Veganism quickly become a "mainstream" diet along with the Keto, for example. However, we can't really put Veganism in the same basket as most of the mainstream diets, as the guidelines here are very well defined and backed up by scientific research, especially when it comes to its benefits to our health and weight loss. Due to its popularity, you are probably already a bit familiar with the concept of the diet, but it's important to highlight some particularities as well. Beginning with, is Veganism a diet, to begin with?

Veganism, for many people, is not a diet but a lifestyle. People can become adepts of Veganism because they want to lose weight, become healthier, or simply because they agree with the concept of the "diet", which means that people can become vegan even if they don't have any concern about their health or weight loss. Being so, it is unfair to resume Veganism to simply a "diet". Nonetheless, what is truthfully Veganism then? And Vegetarianism? Many people confuse the two diets and believe they are synonymous. Other people simply assume that Veganism is very difficult to follow. However, the two diets fit within the same "umbrella" but are ultimately different. Still, they are more manageable and simpler to follow than you might think.

The concept of Veganism

Veganism is defined as the lifestyle that seeks to eliminate any and all consumption of items produced both directly and indirectly using animal materials. Basically, vegans do not buy any item that causes animals to suffer, directly or indirectly. This philosophy is not limited to food, so we cannot just call it a "diet". Vegans do not buy or use leather, products tested on animals such as shampoos and beauty items, and any item that might have any animal resource.

Even food items that theoretically do not cause suffering to animals during their production, such as honey, are also eliminated from the diet. The reason is that vegans believe that animals should not be used, under any circumstances, for our service. This includes being used as food, entertainment, resource, tool, research, and experiments, and sometimes as a pet.

Does this mean that the only reason someone might have to become vegan will always be the animal cause or environmental issues? Not necessarily! Some vegans, such as me, also consider the diet healthier and more efficient for weight loss. Being so, choosing the vegan lifestyle allows me to stick to a diet that is not only beneficial for the environment and animals but also for my health, which is important as both causes are dear to my heart. These are some of the standard guidelines:

What can I and cannot eat?

The foods that you must remove from your vegan diet are every single product that might contain animal resources. You might also be mindful of your everyday products with similar resources or tested in animals. That is if you want to expand Veganism to other areas of your life. Primarily, when it comes to dieting, you must stay away from the following:

The Ultimate Vegan and Intermittent Fasting Guide

- Any type of meat (Beef, Lamb, Pork, and other red meats)
- Duck, Chicken, and other poultry.
- Fish and shellfish (Clams, Mussels, Crabs, etc.)
- Eggs.
- Cheese, Butter.
- Honey.
- Milk, Ice Cream, Cream, any other dairy products.
- Mayonnaise.
- Any ingredient or item that comes from animal cruelty.

Does it sound like you are left without any other option to eat? Quite the opposite. Even after removing animal products, you are still left with countless possibilities to create your meal plan. This is what a common vegan grocery list might look like:

The Ultimate Vegan and Intermittent Fasting Guide

Vegetables	Fruits	Snacks & Sweets	Flavour	Staples	Proteins	Pantry
Artichoke	Apple	Dried Fruit	Olive Oil	Quinoa	Almonds	Canned Coconut Milk
Asparagus	Apricots	Popcorn Kernels	Coconut Oil	Rice	Walnuts	Almond Milk
Beetroot	Avocado	Coconut Flakes	Sesame Oil	Millet	Pecans	Soy Milk
Bell Pepper	Banana	Shredded Coconut	Peanut Oil	Barley	Pistachios	Rice Milk
Broccoli	Blackberries	Vegan Chocolate Chips	Veggie Stock	Oats	Pumpkin Seeds	
Brussels Sprout	Blueberries	Vegan Cookies	Capers	Granola	Sunflower Seeds	
Cabbage	Cantaloupe	Dark Chocolate	Olives	Cereals	Almond Butter	
Carrot	Cherries		Rice Vinegar	Chips	Peanut Butter	
Cauliflower	Coconut Meat		Balsamic Vinegar	Crackers	Sunflower Butter	
Celery	Cranberries		Turmeric	Vegan Mac & Cheese	Raw Cashews	
Corn	Figs		Sweeteners	Canned Soups	Chickpeas	
			Soy Sauce	Vegan Pasta options	Black beans	
			Sriracha	Vegan Bread		

The Ultimate Vegan and Intermittent Fasting Guide

Cucumber	Grapefruit		Tahini		Pinto Beans	
Eggplant	Grapes		White Miso		Lentils	
Green bean	Guava		Maple Syrup		Plant-Based Protein Powder	
Lettuce	Jackfruit		Hummus			
	Kiwi				Tofu	
Mushrooms	Lemon				Tempeh	
Onion	Lime				Tofurkey	
Pea	Mandarin					
Potato	Mango					
Pumpkin	Nectarine					
Radish	Orange					
Sweet Potato	Papaia					
Tomato	Pear					
Zucchini	Peaches					
Leafy Greens	Pitaya					
	Pineapple					

	Plums					
	Strawberries					
	Tangerine					
	Watermelon					

Due to the popularity of the vegan diet, you won't have problems finding restaurants or cafés that offer vegan food options. Even if you are unable to find vegan options on the menu initially, most of them are ready to make any changes that you might request, such as removing the meat from your salad, for example. Being so, you don't have to worry about stopping to eat your favourite dishes. There is also a vegan version for almost every single thing that you might enjoy, such as pizza, bread, cookies, cakes, etc.

Is Veganism healthy, and will I automatically lose weight?

Some people believe that Veganism is a very complex and not so healthy diet. This is understandable because the label "vegan" on a product doesn't necessarily mean that the product in question is healthy. Quite the contrary, there are countless vegan junk food options that can be equally unhealthy. This means that it is entirely possible to be fully vegan and still follow an unhealthy diet, which will prevent you from losing weight. These are some of the common vegan junk foods you might find. Keep in mind that most of these products are "accidentally" vegan, meaning it just so happens that they don't have any animal ingredients:

- Cinnamon Life
- Duncan Hines Chewy Fudge Brownie Mix
- SkinnyPop White Cheddar Flavoured Popped Popcorn
- Airheads
- Cracker Jack
- Doritos Spicy Sweet Chili-Flavoured Tortilla Chips
- Fritos
- Fruit by the Foot
- Kettle Brand Potato Chips
- Lay's Potato Chips

- Nature Valley Crunchy Granola Bars
- Ritz Crackers
- Ruffles Original Potato Chips
- Sour Patch Kids
- Wheat Thins
- Hershey's Syrup
- Ore Ida Tater Tots
- Pringles
- Nabisco Oreo
- Jell-O Cook & Serve Vanilla Pudding & Pie Filling

Aside from processed junk food that might be vegan, such as the listed above, it is also entirely possible to get vegan junk food in fast food places or even make your own at home. For example, French Fries are vegan, but they are far from being healthy and can get in the way of your weight loss process. While preparing any food at home, you might also add too much sodium, for example, which is also bad for your health. You might also use sources of trans fat to prepare your meals, which will increase your calorie consumption and is also not ideal for those who want to lose weight. Being so, if your goal with the diet is to lose weight, simply staying away from animal products isn't enough. You must be mindful of what you eat within this category of foods as well. Better yet, if you are careful about other mistakes that you might make on your diet that might prevent you from losing weight, you will get even better results. We'll discuss them in chapter 08.

Chapter 05. Intermittent Fasting Guidelines

Many people looking for more information about intermittent Fasting are faced with this central question: "Why is fasting better than diets"? There is a belief that anything that deviates from the essential dietary recommendations for weight loss, such as "you must eat every three hours" in order to boost your metabolism or "Just eat less and exercise more", won't work. These guidelines are outdated, and there are plenty of new studies being released every day to prove they are wrong.

The problem is that the damage is done. These basic recommendations have led the United States to the biggest obesity crisis in history! This is massive because it simply does not match with what we see on T.V. and social media. While it seems that people are often even more concerned about their health and fitness, we are becoming bigger. As I have said at the beginning of this material, this shows that clearly, the conventional method does not work. Instead, it only leads adults to stress, hunger, and the yoyo effect. Therefore, to understand and accept the Intermittent Fasting Guidelines, we need to break free from everything you think we know about dieting, weight loss, and healthy eating.

Temporary Solution versus a Lifestyle change

A significant factor that differentiates the conventional dieting method from Fasting is that there is a belief that diets are temporary. You must agree with me on this. How many times did you start a diet, thinking you are going to follow its guidelines for the rest of your life? Probably never. Instead, whenever you start a diet, you choose the one that promises you the best and quickest results. You are then willing to deprive yourself of foods you like solely to lose weight – No health concerns here - while thinking that you can simply "end" the diet and go back to your old eating habits once you reach your goal weight. Then, you gain all the weight back.

When it comes to Fasting, this possibility does not exist. Or, at the very least, things are less likely to go down this path. Fasting is not a temporary method that restricts what you consume. You can and should fast even after reaching your desired weight. You might also keep fasting whenever you can, even if you don't want to lose weight, to begin with, simply for its health benefits. Fasting guidelines are extremely easy to follow. They also offer a lot of flexibility, as you will soon see, which decreases the chances that you will fall into "temptation". Looking exclusively at the intermittent fasting guidelines, you can eat whatever you want during your daily eating window. The difference is that here, we will also follow the Vegan guidelines we discussed in the previous chapter.

Nonetheless, while following both strategies, I could still go out with friends to a bar or restaurant. I could still have dinner with friends and have get-togethers at my house. Fasting never felt like a task for me, but rather as a regular part of my life. When you get used to the cycles, it becomes almost part of your routine, and you will catch yourself fasting even without the intent of doing so, especially since you will notice drastic changes in your appetite. Following the basic guidelines, however, you can start by fasting for a few hours every day. Best of all, you will be the one to decide on how many hours you will fast and in which part of your day you will place these hours. That is, if you want to start fasting at 7 AM, you can. If you're going to start fasting at 7 PM, you can as well. The control is in your hands. Still, people who begin practising Fasting will usually follow one of these four cycles:

Intermittent Fasting Schedule

As we mentioned earlier, these pre-established fasting schedules or cycles are used by most Intermittent Fast supporters. They are:

- 12 hours of Fasting (eating window of 12 hours)
- 14 hours of Fasting (eating window of 10 hours)
- 16 hours of Fasting (eating window of 8 hours)
- 24 hours of Fasting (24 hours of Fasting followed by a typical fasting day of 12, 14, or 16 hours)
- Alternative Fasting (24 hours of fasting every other day. You fast for 14 hours and then have an eating window of 24 hours)

It is essential for you to know that the hours of sleep also count as Fasting. That is, suppose you decide to fast for 12 hours every day during your first week of intermittent Fasting, with Fasting beginning at 8 PM and ending at 8 AM. In this case, you just fasted for 12 hours in a simple way in which you spent the majority of the time sleeping. If you decide to fast for 16 hours, you can do the same. In this case, think of a Fasting cycle starting at 8 PM and ending at 12 PM the next day. As you can see, the process of Fasting is actually quite simple, flexible, without mysteries, and very easy to follow.

You can also rotate and modify cycles according to your hunger. For example, let's say you decided to fast for 16 hours, but after you reached 12 hours of Fasting, you received an invitation for dinner that just seems like too good of an opportunity to miss. You want to hang out with your friends and have a good time. In that case, you can end your fast earlier at the 12 o'clock mark. On the other hand, suppose you decide to fast for 14 hours, but you noticed that you are not even hungry yet when you hit the mark. In that case, you can extend your fasting cycle by an additional 2 hours to complete the 16 hours fasting cycle, or even 24 hours, depending on how hungry you are. It all depends on your hunger cues. Intermittent Fasting means freedom and control.

How to start fasting

If you want to start fasting to lose weight or become healthier, you must do it slowly so that your body won't be put in a sudden state of stress. Both your body and mind must have the chance to adapt, mainly because there will be some initial side effects of Fasting, which we will discuss later in this book. However, to start following the cycles listed in this chapter, you can use some of these tips that helped me during my journey. Initially, these are the rules you must abide by:

- Simplified Fasting: During fasting hours, you can only consume water (sparkling or regular), unsweetened black coffee, and unsweetened tea. Therefore, Fasting does not mean not consuming **any** food whatsoever, but only drinking water, tea or coffee without sugar as much and whenever you want.

- Simplified Dieting: During your eating window every day, it is crucial that you do not attempt to eat more in order to compensate for the fasting hours. The goal is that you are able to eat normally, just as you would if you were not fasting. No more and no less. For example, if you are going to fast from 7 PM until 9 AM, you can have breakfast and lunch normally and according to your hunger. Don't try to add other unnecessary meals just because you "can" eat during these hours. Don't try to increase your meal size either. Follow your hunger cues, and even if they might be all over the place initially due to hormonal imbalance, if you push through the first few days of Fasting, you will notice that it becomes easier and more manageable.

- Fasting cycles are flexible: As you saw, there are many pre-determined cycles that you can choose from, but be aware that these same cycles are flexible. For example, again, if you fast from 7 PM to 9 AM but wake up at 7 AM and feel really hungry by 8 AM, you can simply have your meal. This can happen primarily when you work outside. If you have a commitment at 9 AM, for example, and you are already hungry, don't push through as you will be unable to eat while you run your errands. In this case, shortening your cycle by one hour is a better option. The important thing is that you at least try to follow the schedules as faithfully as possible.

- Which days of the week should you choose to fast? You can do intermittent Fasting every day of the week, or three times a week, four times a week ... The choice is entirely yours. However, do not exceed 24 hours of uninterrupted Fasting. That is, if you fast an entire Monday for the next day, fast for less time, 12 hours, 14 or 16, but do not complete 48 hours of Fasting. Let's say you start your fast at 12 PM on a Monday and end it at 12 PM on Tuesday. Then, ensure that you start your eating window by that time. If you fast every day, in this case, you should have an eating window of at least 8 hours, starting your fasting cycle again by 8 PM.

The Ultimate Vegan and Intermittent Fasting Guide

I'm not saying that the process will be a ride at the park, but I do find that following Intermittent Fasting guidelines was easier than most of the diets and methods that I had tried in the past. To make it easier for you, I will provide a one-week intermittent fasting sample that you can use by the end of this chapter. Once you do try to start your cycles, however, you can use these tips to ensure a smooth transition:

- Adaptation: Skip a meal: How about starting the day without breakfast? Upon waking up, you can consume some of the foods allowed during Fasting (coffee, tea, and water) and have lunch and dinner as usual. Or you can have typical meals during the day and skip dinner. This will promote an adaptation to Fasting and make the process simpler and more familiar.
- Brush your teeth: During the first few days of fasting or during the adaptation phase mentioned above, you may feel like eating during your fasting hours. Not because you are hungry, but because you have the habit/routine of eating around that time. When you brush your teeth, it

sends a subliminal signal to the brain that you have just eaten since you also routinely brush your teeth at the end of a meal.

- Forget schedules: During Fasting or during the adaptation phase, try to ignore socially determined times for meals. Our body does not have clocks. You "feel like eating" at noon because you created a routine where you eat every day at that same time. Suppose you decided to skip breakfast during the adaptation phase, surprisingly, "lunch time" arrived, and you are not hungry, but you choose to eat because "it is lunch time". Break this paradigm. Eat only when you are hungry.

The Ultimate Vegan and Intermittent Fasting Guide

One-Week Intermittent Fasting Sample

Sunday	Monday	Tuesday	Wednesday	Thursday	Friday	Saturday
Eating Window from 8 AM to 8 PM	Eating Window from 8 AM to 8 PM	Eating Window from 10 AM to 8 PM	Eating Window from 10 AM to 8 PM	Eating Window from 12 PM to 8 PM	Eating Window from 12 PM to 8 PM	Eating Window from 02 PM to 8 PM
(12 hours eating window)	(12 hours eating window)	(10 hours eating window)	(10 hours eating window)	(08 hours eating window)	(08 hours eating window)	(06 hours eating window)

Chapter 06. Benefits of Intermittent Fasting & Vegan Diet

The Perfect Weight Loss Combo

The systems in which Fasting and the vegan diet can help with weight loss vary. Besides helping reduce your hunger and Ghrelin levels, Fasting additionally supports weight loss by promoting a calorie deficit. You need energy to do every single thing, even breathing. Being so, your body will need thousands of calories just to keep your organs functioning. This number of calories is called a B.M.R. – Basal Metabolic Rate. When we add our workout routine, our work, our study section, our B.M.R. increases until we reach a new total. Then, you must obtain these calories through consuming foods as they are sources of macronutrients. There are three of them. Proteins have five calories per gram, and so do carbohydrates. On the other hand, fats are the macros with the highest energy value, carrying nine calories per gram.

Knowing your B.M.R. is essential because this number is directly connected to weight loss. At the end of the day, you need to eat fewer calories than you burn on a daily basis if you want to lose weight. This should happen throughout your entire weight loss journey, and when it doesn't, people become stuck. You know, those two or three last kilos that you can't seem to lose. As you lose weight, your B.M.R. changes as well, which is why you must always keep this number in mind.

You lose weight when you enter a calorie deficit, which essentially means burning more calories than you consume. If you do the opposite and consume more calories than you need, your body will convert them into triglycerides and store them in your adipose tissue. Every time you consume more calories than you need, your fat deposits slowly increase, and if you keep repeating the cycle for many days and even months, you will gain a considerable amount of weight. To ensure that you are consuming fewer calories than you burn, however, you must first find out how many calories your body demands every day. This will vary depending on your routine. The busier you are, the more calories you will burn. For example, if you are a sedentary person, your daily calorie demand will usually stay on the lower side, which will make exceeding your calories much easier. Although it's challenging to find out precisely the number of calories you burn every day just to stay alive, online BMR calculators can give an estimate that might be helpful during your weight loss process.

The perfect approach, in our case, is to find out the B.M.R. and implement a fasting method along with changes in your diet. As long as you are eating a healthier diet along with Fasting, your results will be much better and happen quicker than if you just fasted. The ideal is that you "spend" your daily calories with nutrient-dense foods such as fruits and vegetables, which will increase your fibre consumption as well. By doing this, we slowly create a new cycle that "attacks" our weight from different sides. Fasting reduces your appetite. You then eat less and use your calories, consuming vegan food options, which increase your fibre consumption and improve your gut health. This aids digestion and supports weight loss. And so on! Eventually, your entire lifestyle will be directed towards your weight loss goal.

Nonetheless, it is essential to highlight that if you fail to follow the proper fasting guidelines described in the previous chapter and spend your daily calories consuming vegan junk food, you will hardly see any results. Although Fasting offers brilliant and promising outcomes with regards to reducing your daily calorie consumption, it is essential that you also do your part in trying to choose the best possible food sources available. You might also make the mistake of purposefully trying to eat more during your eating windows and buying a lot of processed vegan foods thinking they are healthy. Try to avoid this habit! Homemade food will offer you more control of the ingredients used in your meals and will often be a much better option than a vegan cake, for example.

At the end of the day, for people who are on a weight loss journey, Fasting can function as an incredible asset to help accomplish your goals in regards to restricting calories simply because you are making your daily window become much smaller. When combined with less appetite, less time to eat should be enough to lead to a calorie deficit naturally. Keep in mind that the standard daily calorie suggestion for most people will stay between 1,800 and 2,200 calories, which means that people tend to base their diets around these numbers. However, each of us has a different routine, and the number of daily calories we need can drastically vary from one person to the other.

Once you have your BMR using the calculator that I provided, which will usually range between 2,000 and 4,000 calories for most people, a majority of you will try to make sure you are eating less than that by counting calories, which seems to be the easiest option here. However, I personally do not like to count calories, as I believe it damages our relationship with foods and is simply a tedious task. Also, counting calories has nothing to do with eating healthy. If you set a limit of 3,000 calories for your day, you can still find ways to fit "unhealthy" food items within this limit, which might make you lose weight, but it is not the healthiest choice. Thus, reducing your calorie intake with Fasting and following a vegan diet is a better choice because it allows you to improve your health while also dropping some weight.

With time, there is a massive chance that you will change your eating habits to a point when you are no longer dependent on following an intermittent fasting cycle or being careful about what you eat. Instead, you will simply eat less as you have become used to it. In this case, even if you have a 24-hour eating window, you will also end up eating fewer calories than you used to before you started to practice Fasting and following a vegan diet.

This will be very helpful as most of the time people have no idea of how much they actually eat, especially as eating is something that they do on a daily basis, multiple times a day. Can you remember how much you ate yesterday? Can you describe your meals in detail? What about the day before? With time, you become more aware of the few meals you do have, making you eat less, even if you have the chance to eat as much as you want. Considering this, Fasting could be a superb strategy not just for a "quick weight loss" but the best option for a healthier lifestyle in the long run too.

There is also the chance that you will simply take Fasting and Veganism with you for life. All things considered, if you are feeling better about yourself, losing weight, and improving your health, why stop? Even after losing four stones, I still fast as it became a part of my life and something that provides countless benefits for both my mental and physical health, and I don't plan on stopping any time soon either. I can guarantee that once you start, you won't want to stop too.

Higher fibre consumption

Fibres are known for being a type of carbohydrate that can't be digestive by the body, which means that any fibre you consume will pass through your digestive system rather slowly, reaching your intestine almost intact, where it will serve as food for the bacteria living in your gut. People following a Vegan diet will usually consume more fibre sources such as vegetables and fruits as they will not consume animal protein. Whole grains such as wild rice are often typical food in vegan diets, which are also packed with fibre.

As fibre passes through your body slowly, it will keep you full for longer. That is one of the main reasons why junk food is bad for your health and causes weight gain, as they tend to pass through your digestive system rather quickly, causing insulin spikes and making you hungry again after just a couple of hours. A diet with more fibre will also improve your gut health, which will further support weight loss as your digestion will improve, and your body will better absorb nutrients.

Faster metabolism for more weight loss

Intermittent Fasting will boost your metabolism primarily thanks to the fact that your norepinephrine levels increase while fasting. This is a neurotransmitter that can make your body burn more fat and thus supports weight loss. As a matter of fact, Fasting is associated with fat burning through many different mechanisms, and studies show that simply fasting for a few weeks, even without any diet changes, can boost your metabolism by up to 8%. When combined with a healthier eating strategy, these results can be even better. However, it is vital to notice that even fasting for shorter amounts of time can lead to positive results. When I started to use Fasting as a method during my weight loss journey, I began with smaller daily cycles. I was afraid of making drastic changes in my diet and not being unable to stick to them for an extended period of time. Gradually, I increased the duration of the cycles but I could already notice positive results even in the first few days while still taking baby steps.

Fasting also helps with calorie reduction as well as supporting more fat burning and pushing for higher levels of important neurotransmitters for weight loss. However, the vital point in question is that you will be able to notice that you are eating fewer calories even without trying to do so. It will merely happen as your eating windows become smaller, and your appetite decreases. On average, people who fast can eat between 500 and 1000 fewer calories every day even if they don't make any changes to their diet. In our case, eating healthier vegan food and following the proper weight-loss guidelines will lead to even better results.

Perhaps, the fact that Fasting can promote more fat burning might be the biggest reason why the method is so effective for weight loss. You know that food is energy, which is called calories, and that each macronutrient has a different number of calories per gram. Whenever you have a meal, you are essentially filling your own fuel tank to allow you to have the energy to move on with your daily tasks. Think of your meals as a moment when you recharge your energy levels. An easier way to understand how this works is by thinking of your body as a machine, a car, or an aeroplane, for example.

When you are running out of fuel, you usually say that your car is running on low, which means that it is using the remaining fuel left (your fat stores), which are only utilized when you are genuinely running out of fuel (when glucose levels are low). Think of it as a reserve, the last resource. The same happens with your body. When you don't provide any fuel (eat), your body will then use that last fuel source to maintain your energy levels (Fat deposits). However, if you are constantly going to the gas station, your tank will always be full, which means your car will never need to run on low fuel, correct? If you are constantly eating and providing more energy to your body, the same happens, and you will never need to use your fat deposits for energy. Instead, they will just keep growing, increasing your fat percentage. The difference here is that although running on low fuel all the time can damage your car, using your fat deposits for fuel is actually your goal. While fasting, you essentially run out of "fresh" glucose. Since you are not eating for a lot of hours, this makes our bodies become extremely efficient in using the fat deposits for energy, which is called entering a stage of Ketosis. The only two dieting strategies that allow this to happen are the Keto Diet and Intermittent Fasting.

A Vegan diet is more nutrient-dense than other options

Since you must eliminate animal products from your diet, you automatically start to consume more fruits, vegetables, whole grains, and vegan protein sources. These foods are packed with nutrients and vitamins necessary for your health and body, which means that you naturally consume more micronutrients when compared to other diets by switching to a vegan diet.

Some examples of this are vitamins A, C, and E. You will also consume more antioxidants, fibre, and other plant compounds that are great for your health. A vegan diet can also be richer in folate – which is excellent for pregnant women, magnesium, potassium, and other minerals. Be mindful, however, that you must also be careful about specific vitamins as well. When not done correctly, a vegan diet can be lower on fatty acids – usually found in fatty fish, and especially vitamin B12. The best approach then is to take Omega-3 and Omega-6 supplements to ensure you are consuming enough of these nutrients, and as for B12, buying nutritional yeast, fortified plant milk, tempeh, mushrooms, and seaweed might help.

A Vegan Diet will lower your blood sugar levels.

When combined with Fasting, this benefit can be even more significant, as you know that Fasting can lower Insulin levels. While you are fasting, you also reduce your sugar intake, which further lowers blood sugar levels. However, a vegan diet can also be beneficial. Vegans tend to have almost 80% less risk of having type 2 diabetes, insulin resistance, and high blood sugar levels.

As a matter of fact, research suggests that a vegan diet can actually be more beneficial in reducing blood sugar levels than the A.D.A. – American Diabetes Association specifically designed diet, as well as the

A.H.A. – American Heart Association, and the NCEP – National Cholesterol Education Program's diets.

Veganism is also directly connected to heart health, as saturated fat – found in animal protein – is often linked to heart diseases. Having a meal plan primarily focused on fruits and vegetables can positively impact your heart health because of the nutritional value of these food options. In general, vegans have about a 75% lower risk of developing high blood pressure, for example.

Since you are consuming less saturated fat and other sources of fat, your lipid profile also improves. This means that your LDL – bad cholesterol – drops. This is vital as LDL can clog your arteries, causing a stroke and other heart complications. Veganism can also reduce your overall cholesterol levels, being most of the time more effective in doing so when compared to other mainstream diets.

Fasting and Veganism – Relationship with Food

Regardless if you want to lose weight or simply improve your health, your relationship to food could be one of the key, if not most important, factors for a permanent, long-term health improvement. As of now, we can list a number of disordered eating behaviours that are crucial in one's relationship with food and its impact on their weight. However, it's fair to admit that the claim that intermittent Fasting alone can cure an unstable eating behaviour or that the fasting system may be helpful in changing your relationship with food on a deeper level can be a bit risky. However, the benefits of the strategy on how you see food, whether it be in a positive or negative light are undeniable.

One of the main reasons why I could not lose weight before is that I could not stick with the same diet. No matter how great I believed the diet was, I still could not do it. Sometimes I could even see some weight loss after a few days, but this still wasn't enough for me to follow the guidelines for more than a couple of weeks. If I tried to, I had these episodes where everything that I wanted was to go back to my old eating habits and eat whatever I wanted in peace. Even while following healthy eating habits and making better choices, it is still difficult to break these habits.

However, it can undoubtedly be expected that Fasting can also be used to change this unhealthy relationship, at least for people who are used to overeating and binge eating very frequently. How does one go about it, then? It is a standard answer given by several healthcare professionals and also by our official Nutritional Guidelines that one needs to eat at all times. However, as we explained earlier in this book, there is no evidence that eating more times a day can impact weight loss. As a matter of fact, we know that Fasting can reduce our appetites, which actually supports weight loss.

The argument that helped make this recommendation so common was that people believed it would trigger a withdrawal reaction if you made someone addicted to food eat fewer times a day. After just a couple of days, you would show complete unwillingness to continue eating healthily and would return to your former eating patterns. They thought that when someone is overweight and unhealthy, they will overlook the fact that they are getting less food if the portions were evenly distributed throughout the day. Thus, eating smaller portions would allow them to keep eating the entire day, even if the overall amount of food was smaller.

The problem with this line of reasoning would be that while this principle was gradually being propagated, there really is no evidence that supports any of it. That being said, it is easy to identify other flaws as well. For instance, the fact that making someone who is addicted to food eat so many times a day would give them countless opportunities to overeat. It's like telling them to think about food all of the time. Thinking about food all of the time is not something natural to us and shouldn't be reinforced. You really do not need to be eating every two hours because this means you will then think about food just as frequently, which is by far not the healthiest lifestyle.

Think about that for a while. The contrast between a compulsive overeater and an alcoholic is that people don't really need to drink beer to stay alive. Thus, it is possible, in fact, to eliminate alcohol altogether from their lives. But when it comes to food, it isn't the same.

We also need to eat, and we can't go weeks, months, or maybe even years without having to eat. As a direct consequence, having to deal with somebody who is addicted to food is a far more challenging task. If we were to use the same reasoning we use for people addicted to drugs, the right approach would be to remove food altogether. As we all know, that's not achievable with food. What should we do then? Tell them to eat all of the time? Every two or three hours?

It feels unhelpful because it is. On the other side of the spectrum, if you were fasting, you wouldn't even have to think about food for a long time throughout the day, which provides a perfect opportunity to stay busy doing other things, such as focusing on your work, friendships, passions, activities, and so on. You don't always have to think about what you'll eat next because you "can't" eat. You're fasting. This enables you to concentrate on other important things and can finally eliminate your food dependency.

Though this component of the fasting benefits is something that has not yet been explored, the suggestion is quite interesting. Many of those who begin to implement a fasting cycle to their routines often notice that food becomes something other than a habit. Still, instead, it becomes a way of caring for their body and providing energy when necessary. Being so, the best way to ensure you will be successful would be to not think about food all of the time and avoid using food to hide your other emotions like happiness, sadness, frustration, etc. Thankfully, Fasting can help you develop the ability to feel these things without running to food.

Intermittent Fasting gave me an opportunity to break free from being emotionally attached to food. Since I could only eat during certain hours of the day, it was simply pointless to keep thinking about my meals during any other time. Like many others who fast, including me, you might realize that your relationship with food dramatically improves, and you do not feel the need to overeat and over-indulge as frequently as before. This can mean not only weight loss in a long-term approach but also improved fitness and a healthier mind and body, which are ultimately the best benefit one could get regardless of their weight loss goals.

Lower Blood Sugar and Insulin Levels

Another way that fasting aids weight loss is by controlling insulin levels. As you know, insulin resistance can lead to weight gain, and the only way to avoid it is to limit your sugar consumption so that it does not overpower your insulin production. This often happens when fasting. Being so, the method has been shown to help control blood sugar levels, preventing Insulin Resistance and thus type 2 diabetes.

In one study[3], three times a day, during the mornings, afternoons, and evenings, patients with type 2 diabetes had their glucose levels self-monitored, and each of them fasted daily. At the end of the study, fasting blood samples were taken, and participants' blood sugar levels were reduced. Several studies have also shown that different types of Fasting, like intuitive Fasting and alternative Fasting, can also prevent insulin resistance.

Because Fasting lowers blood sugar levels, the pancreas will release less Insulin to remove glucose from the bloodstream and store it in the cells. This improves Insulin resistance and regulates the levels of this hormone. However, please note that most studies have shown us that women will often see better results than men, so if you are a male, you might notice that the progress might happen at a slower pace. Still, the truth of the matter is that Fasting is still an effective strategy to control Insulin levels.

By doing so, your body can prevent insulin resistance and type 2 diabetes and enhance glucose to energy efficiency, reduce insulin spikes, and reduce cravings and fat storage in the adipose tissue. This supports weight loss and improves your chances of successfully reaching your goals.

Sharpening your senses with Fasting

Usually, one of the main arguments used by those who are against Fasting or those who are afraid of the practice is that our brain needs glucose to function. By Fasting, you drastically reduce your glucose levels for a few hours, which in theory, would not be good for your brain health as the organ can only use this one source of fuel to have energy. Being so, the myth that Fasting is harmful to brain health has become a common reason for many people to avoid the method.

In this debate, while some people believe that Fasting can be great for brain health, others believe it can be dangerous. I can tell you straight away that the first option is correct but that, in fact, your brain needs glucose to function. Thus, we can affirm that your body needs glucose and that Fasting is beneficial, as both sentences are correct.

Let's discuss one at a time. Yes, your brain does need glucose. This is the reason why people are often against the Keto Diet – as the main principle of the diet is to shift the body's fuel source – and Intermittent Fasting. Since you spend more hours without eating, your glucose levels drastically drop, which would technically deplete your brain of energy.

It is true that the brain is the only part of the body that relies solely on glucose, which means that without any glucose, the brain will suffer serious harm. Nonetheless, this shouldn't actually be a reason for concern, as you actually do eat while fasting. A fasting cycle with intermittent Fasting will last, at most, 24 hours. Most of them are usually even shorter than that. There were probably multiple instances throughout your life when you fasted for just as long as a fasting cycle without even noticing, whether because you were too busy or you overslept, for example. The reason doesn't matter. The critical point is that you are less dependent on food than you might think.

Your body doesn't truly shut down when you are sleeping, correct? All of your organs are still very much functioning, and many important processes will exclusively happen during your sleep. Hormonal regulation, for example, often occurs when you reach R.E.M. sleep. This means that your body is still using energy, including your brain, even while you are sleeping. But you are not really eating, and your glucose levels are down as well. This essentially means that your body is highly effective in using its own resources to provide energy when you are not eating, and we can go much longer without providing any glucose to our brains through our dietary choices. As soon as your fasting cycle ends, you will eat, as usual, so your brain will never go more than a few hours without a new batch of glucose.

The other crucial aspect is that although our brain does need glucose, thankfully for us, our body is a magnificent and powerful machine, which ensures that anything that is so important for your body to work correctly will not be entirely dependent on your dietary choices. When you go for hours without food, the body produces glucose for your brain on its own. As a matter of fact, the body does this when you sleep at night as well. This is made possible by what is called "gluconeogenesis", a mechanism that will break down proteins and turn them into glucose for the brain to use when you are not providing sugar sources through your meals.

If we know that Fasting isn't harmful to the brain, could it be the opposite? Could it be that Fasting is actually not only harmless but also beneficial? To discuss this side of the spectrum, we have a lot of scientific research to discuss in order to prove these claims. We can also observe how other animals deal with the Fasting's dilemma and how they can survive without having access to a supermarket or 24-hour delivery service. In the wild, a lioness, which is responsible for hunting and providing food for her cubs and for the lions in her pride, will often go days without finding a proper prey to hunt. When she finds it and successfully takes it down, she, the lion, and the cubs will freely eat as much as they can and then again go days without having another prey. The main factor here is that during these moments, when she can't find prey and her family is starving, she needs to have sharper senses in order to hunt. If Fasting made her weak and lethargic, she would essentially fail to take down any prey and would eventually starve. We are animals too, and the principle is the same with us. When fasting, our senses become sharper, we are able to focus better, and our cognitive abilities improve.

Being so, it comes as no surprise that, according to studies, our brain can actually work better when fasting, with enhanced cognitive function, reasoning skills, memory, and alertness. These are characteristics needed for an animal to hunt, and the body significantly improves them during Fasting. Research with mice demonstrated that animals that were subjected to intermittent Fasting every couple of days grew stronger than those that were not. Thus, Fasting was established as an essential factor that improves the physical efficiency of mice!

This occurs because a protein known as BDNF – Brain-Derived Neurotrophic Factor – is released in more significant quantities during Fasting. This protein has been linked to learning and memory and stimulating the development of new nerve cells in the hippocampus. Furthermore, BDNF has been shown to make neurons in our brains more resistant to stress.

Another critical mechanism that occurs during Fasting is called "autophagy", which is the removal of damaged molecules. This prevents defective mitochondria from growing and expanding. The theory is that our bodies are conserving nutrients while fasting, which will then be used to boost growth once you eat again. As a long-term consequence, these on and off mechanisms will potentially strengthen memory, learning processes, and make the brain more responsive to stress.

These fasting benefits to brain health can be further proved by the fact that, initially, Fasting was used to cure brain disorders in addition to being used as a method for spiritual development. Like the Keto diet, Fasting was used as a treatment method for epilepsy in the twentieth century. Ancient Greek doctors recommended the procedure to treat this and many other health issues. Hippocrates also advocated for the use of Fasting as an epilepsy remedy, and the practice eventually became almost standard practice for treating similar conditions.

Fasting was tested for its effectiveness in treating such conditions in 1991, and the findings revealed that patients who fasted had fewer seizures and fewer side effects from the conditions. Hugh Conklin, a psychiatrist, began to prescribe fasting to epileptic patients in the same year in order to suppress their seizures. He achieved a 50% success rate in adults and a 90% success rate in children using this approach. Fasting, which has long been used to treat epilepsy, has shown excellent brain health and cognitive function outcomes.

Researchers were able to quantify improvements in brain functions and important benefits to brain structures by following a fasting regimen in a study conducted with mice. Fasting can also maintain brain health and increase the development of new nerve cells, which would improve cognitive performance even further. People who fast on a regular basis report improvement in their ability to focus and concentrate, which is something I experienced first-hand when I started fasting.

This occurs because our brain perceives fasting to be a daunting situation. If you are fasting, your brain recognizes that you do not have access to food, so you will need to become "wiser", and in other words, you will have to be more attentive, assertive, and have improved problem-solving abilities in order to obtain food. Thus, your subconscious will automatically be in a proactive mode to make that happen. This also demonstrates why you become far more resistant to stress since your brain understands that not eating can be a stressful condition in and of itself.

To put it simply, if you fast, your brain will not experience any damages. In fact, this will have the inverse result. Fasting improves brain health by making you stronger, sharper, more responsive, and aware and enhances the development of more neurons in your brain, which boosts the connections between them.

The Ultimate Vegan and Intermittent Fasting Guide

Thus, we now know that the myth that lower levels of glucose could damage your brain is fully debunked since evidence has shown that your body is more than capable of making enough glucose for your brain, which is a natural process that occurs when you sleep, and in other situations when you couldn't eat for some reason.

Despite efforts to dismiss Fasting as an effective method for changing and improving your health, academic data suggests the opposite, connecting Fasting to health enhancement and benefits that extend beyond weight loss. Since Fasting was what our ancestors naturally did back in the day, and something that the majority of animals still do when they don't have enough food, it is safe to say that our bodies understood that during Fasting we had to become an improved and more alert version of ourselves, which is an advantage that we can have nowadays by doing shortened fasts than our ancestors and without having to lose all of our modern privileges.

Chapter 07. Side effects of Fasting

Because any changes in your diet are challenging and demand time for the body to fully adapt, certain side effects of following a Vegan Diet and intermittent Fasting will eventually occur. Since I went through this myself, I want to be honest and prepare you for all things related to weight loss and diet so you can start while being completely equipped for anything that you might feel, especially in the first few days of Fasting. So, in this chapter, I shall speak in-depth about some things that people don't talk about weight loss and food that I was able to experience during my own journey that can help you during yours.

Keto Diet? No! Keto Flu? Yes!

The Keto Flu is perhaps the most common side effect of the Keto Diet. But wait, we are not really following the Keto Diet, right? After all, the principles of Veganism and the Keto Diet are entirely opposite to each other. Nonetheless, you will experience the Keto-Flu while fasting, because as you might know, the diet is called as such since your body enters a stage of Ketosis - when the fuel source shifts from glucose to fats. The critical point is that following the Keto Diet isn't the only way to achieve Ketosis. You will also enter this state while fasting; thus, why you might also have the flu during your first few cycles. Keto-flu symptoms are like flu, as the name implies, but you won't have a fever.

Researchers don't know why the flu occurs, but it usually appears after two or three days during fasting cycles, and it is expected that it will naturally disappear once your body adapts to your new routine. Few authors speculated that keto-flu, which is quite common, is nothing but signs of a sugar withdrawal. Several reports actually reveal how sugar is almost as addictive as opioids and nicotine, which makes sense. As we know, glucose activates neurotransmitters in the brain connected to pleasure. Admittedly, Keto-Flu becomes the perfect excuse to stop fasting, but you really shouldn't. If you push through the first few days, the symptoms will disappear by themselves. I'll also provide you with some tips that helped me make the symptoms go away when I was starting my weight loss journey. The Keto-flu symptoms are:

- Diarrheal
- Difficulty sleeping
- Irritability
- Muscle Cramps
- Nausea
- Poor concentration
- Stomach pain
- Sugar cravings
- Weakness

Even if there isn't anything you can do to prevent Keto Flu entirely, you can aim to lower discomfort by paying close attention to several factors. A wise decision is to drink lots of fluids. Many studies suggest that while dieting – and especially fasting, you seem to lose a large amount of water since glycogen connects to the fluids in our bodies, and when the moment arises to be using glycogen as a fuel source, all of the water in the cells will be released from the body. As a result, you must replace all of the water you lose to reduce fatigue and alleviate muscle pain and nausea.

You should also ease up on your training for the first few days of Intermittent Fasting. High-intensity exercises involve a great deal of energy from the body. Going to the gym when your organism is still adjusting to the new energy source can reduce efficiency and cause muscle spasms and abdominal pain. You should still workout, but strive to stick to relatively "easier" activities like biking and walking. I enjoyed walking a lot during my journey, and I learned that it helped me to achieve wonderful results. You should also aim to change your sleep schedule to help minimize irritability. When you can't sleep, your stress hormone levels – cortisol – might increase. Cortisol can also cause weight gain, so be mindful of that.

You might get constipated.

Although you usually consume more fibres on a vegan diet, Fasting can still make you constipated in the first few days. Since you are eating less food, you will go to the bathroom less often. Also, if you are not mindful about how much fibre you are consuming and how much water you are drinking, this can further worsen the symptom. Ensure that these ingredients are found in abundance in your diet: Whole Grains, Leafy Greens, Vegetables, Fruits with the peel. Also, ensure that you are always carrying a water bottle so you can better control how much fluid you are consuming. Most people should drink about two litres of water per day, so if you fill four 500ml bottles and try to finish all of them by the end of the day, then you will have reached your daily goal. Having the bottles in your fridge allows you to understand better how much water you have left for the day.

Electrolytes Imbalance

Electrolyte imbalance would be another known side effect of Intermittent Fasting. You see, aside from controlling your blood sugar levels, Insulin is also responsible for maintaining your sodium levels. When you fast, Insulin's levels drop, and so will your sodium levels. In this case, your body will lose way too many minerals along with the water weight. This can lead to many symptoms that are very similar to those you will experience with the Keto-flu. Some of them are:

- Constipation
- Difficulty sleeping
- Fatigue
- Irregular heartbeat
- Lethargy
- Nausea

Although the symptoms are similar, they are not the same. This means that you can have the Keto-Flu even if you manage to successfully replace all of the sodium that you are losing. Nonetheless, you can do that by adding more salt to your meals. In this case, you don't really need to worry about hypertension or other health consequences of sodium, as you are simply replacing all of the electrolytes you are losing. You might also drink electrolyte-infused water, which is an excellent option since you can still drink it during your fasting hours. Making sure that your electrolytes are replaced will make your first few fasting cycles much more comfortable.

Variation in energy levels

Several people, including me, report feeling energized as a result of Fasting. That being said, this was far from the truth in the first few days. On the contrary! I could feel a decline in energy levels and could barely keep up with my everyday tasks. However, this only lasted for a few days, when my body was still adapting to using fat as fuel during my fasting hours, but what helped was taking it slow during the first few fasting cycles. Occasionally, I could still feel bursts of energy throughout the day. Then, I would quickly try to finish as many tasks as possible, making the best out of my energy. No need to say that after a few days doing daily fasting cycles, my energy levels not only went back to normal but considerably improved.

Chapter 08. The Weight Loss Tips that made me lose four stones

"Coffee can truly become an ally".

Adding a bit more coffee to your routine as a weight loss strategy is often an overlooked strategy. However, you would be surprised to learn that caffeine is one of the most efficient food items to speed up our metabolism. Even more surprisingly, it can boost your metabolism more than water. Research suggests that caffeine can boost your metabolism by up to 30% when you drink it before meals. This is hugely beneficial, as a higher metabolism will make your body burn more calories even while you are resting.

Being so, any method that can successfully lead your body to use your fat deposits will be more than welcomed on your weight loss strategy. Consuming more caffeine, as stated, is one of the most efficient methods of doing so. Other alternatives are, of course, drinking more water and green tea, with the second also containing caffeine but in lesser amounts. Regardless of which drink you choose, try to consume either in its iced version or hot, as both are also thermogenic, which further pushes for fat burning.

Stay away from the "healthy processed" food options

We all know that processed foods are not ideal for our health. Most of the time, these foods are rich in additives, preservatives, food dyes, and more, which are added to maintain flavour, texture, colour, and increase a product's shelf life. In addition to having ingredients that you shouldn't be consuming, these products usually have lower nutritional value, which means they don't really have a lot of nutrients to offer. Being so, when you are trying to lose weight, trying to prepare most of your meals at home or at least reduce the number of processed foods you consume will make a huge difference.

In general, you should buy more ingredients, rather than ready-to-eat meals. By nourishing your body with the vitamins and nutrients it needs, all of your body systems will improve, including your natural detox system responsible for eliminating toxins that can cause hormonal imbalance, which, as you know, can lead to weight gain. By doing so, you won't need to worry about drastically reducing your calorie intake. You will also lose weight thanks to the fact that you're consuming foods that can prevent bloating, improve your digestion, boost your metabolism, and enhance your natural detox system.

Trick your brain into thinking you are not on a diet

This is a proven fact. Our brain does not like diets. This can be explained by several reasons, with one of them simply being sugar addiction. If your brain is addicted to glucose, reducing them from your diet will, of course, cause withdrawal symptoms, which will make following the rules of any diet much more difficult. Being so, as soon as our cravings increase, we quickly run to the first cookie we can find. Another trigger for your brain might be your plate of food. Your brain does not like the idea of reducing the number of calories you are consuming because it fears that it will run out of energy.

Being so, the visual of a half-empty plate might trigger cravings. To avoid this from happening, it is necessary to "trick" the brain. The idea is to focus on volume, not amount. A larger plate will be able to hold more food, correct? By eating on a smaller plate, you can still fill your entire plate with food, giving your brain the visual stimulus that you are eating in abundance while still eating less food. You can also start platting by adding a bed of leaves. This means adding a salad to the bottom of your plate to serve as a base and then place the other ingredients on top. This will give the impression of a full plate, but you are still consuming fewer calories per meal since most of it is still a low-calorie salad.

Cooking your meals will always be the best option.

Temptations are one of the most common issues for people trying to lose weight. Of course, we can't just give up our social lives and avoid going out to eat at some point. However, it is preferable if these are one-time occurrences rather than a dietary pattern. Preparing your meals for the week is an intelligent way to stop dining out or succumbing to a habit of frequent snacking. You'll have more control over the amount of each nutrient in your meals, as well as the number of calories you consume. Furthermore, planning your meals will almost certainly save you money as people usually spend hundreds of dollars on takeout every month. Pick a day, preferably one where you have a lot of free time, to plan out at least your critical meals for the next seven days.

Change your snacking habits.

It is very common for us not to have time to eat meals at the proper times because of our daily work and activities. So, as the hours' pass, we can end up hungry before our next meal, and snacking can help us hold on until we get home to eat, for example. The problem, however, is that we often choose the wrong type of foods to eat when snacking, meaning options that will only make us hungrier. Usually, we turn to fruits, but they aren't always as filling as we would like, and they don't always satisfy us. Protein-dense snacks are the best choice. Proteins have a more considerable satiety power as they are digested slower. Since we are following a vegan diet, having a vegan protein source with us might be difficult. In this case, we can snack on fat sources, such as nuts and seeds. They are also digested slower and will be better than eating fruit.

Don't allow food to dominate your life.

Many obese people have a much more complicated relationship with food than others. It's almost like an addiction, where people can't stop thinking about food. Furthermore, the person may turn to food in extreme situations, whether when they are happy or sad, believing that they should eat to celebrate a good situation or to console themselves in a sad situation. Although professional help may be required for these individuals, you can begin with the basics. Spending several hours just thinking about food is not a good idea. This may be a difficult task in and of itself. As a result, filling your time with activities you enjoy will be a good alternative. Even better if this activity requires calorie expenditure. Consider returning to the dance classes you took as a kid. Alternatively, why not join a book club? Make an effort to fill your mind and time with healthy activities that will benefit both your body and mind.

Move, even if at home.

We know that weight training is not always something that those wanting to lose weight desire to do. Physical activity habits, in general, are often more challenging to maintain than most diets. It is true that food plays a much larger role in weight loss, accounting for roughly 80% of the equation. Physical activities, on the other hand, can be an effective tool for speeding up results. You don't have to spend hours upon hours at the gym; simply make an effort to move. You can buy a yoga mat and do activities at home by watching a youtube video. You'll have no excuse to skip your workout section if you don't even need to leave the house in order to do it. To lose weight faster, try not only to eat fewer calories but also to burn more calories.

The Shortened Guide You Might Need…

Throughout the reading of this book, you received a huge deal of information, so it is understandable if you are confused, not knowing exactly what you should be doing. In short, what are the guidelines you should follow? If you must, print this chapter and have it with you to serve as a constant guide for using both Veganism and Fasting for weight loss.

Vegan Guidelines

- Avoid consuming animal protein and food products that contain animal resources, such as those with milk and eggs as ingredients.
- Try to have vegetables as fruits as the base of every meal, especially to ensure that you are consuming enough fibre.
- Watch out for supplements you might need to take, such as Omega-3 and Vitamin B12.
- Try to cook most of your foods at home so you can have better control of your ingredients.
- Avoid "vegan" junk food such as French fries, Oreos, etc. They are rich in calories and sugar and can prevent weight loss.
- Drink a lot of fluids, including water, coffee, and tea.

Intermittent Fasting Guidelines

- Choose one of the main four cycles to start fasting. Some options are 12, 14, 16, 18 and 24

hours of Fasting. All of the cycles include your sleeping hours.
- While fasting, you can only drink water, coffee, and tea without sugar, as well as electrolyte-infused water.
- Pay extra attention to how much water you are drinking to avoid constipation.
- Be mindful of the Keto-Flu and Electrolyte Imbalance. Consuming just a bit more sodium might help.
- You can fast every day, every other day, or three times a week. It's up to you.
- Keep in mind that fasting cycles can be flexible, and you should listen to your hunger cues.

Overall Weight Loss Tips

- Make sure that you are moving, even if at home. Try to do some online workout classes, but do take it easy during the first few days since you will have less energy.
- Food is an important part of your life, but it shouldn't dominate who you are. Use your time

doing what you like instead of thinking about your next meal.

- Eat on a smaller plate or always add a portion of salad to your plate before adding the remaining ingredients to your meal.
- Coffee can boost your metabolism, so don't be afraid of drinking it.
- Try to stay away from "processed" vegan or dieting products. They are not healthy and will often have countless harmful chemicals in their formula.

What made the most difference to me was being able to disconnect a little bit from food and spend my time focusing on other things. Fasting helped me with that, and I'm sure it is a habit that I will never let go of. I'm also still a vegan, even after losing four stones, and I don't plan on going back to eat meat whatsoever. I'm aware that my current eating pattern is what made me lose weight, to begin with, so I have no intention of making the mistake of going back to my usual ways. Better yet, I'm not even tempted to do so. Fasting allows me freedom and helps me be in control of what I eat, and following the vegan guidelines is also easy and enjoyable.

I hope that with the information I provided in this book, you are able to start your new weight loss/health journey and that you will achieve success. The most important thing is to be comfortable and happy with yourself, regardless of the number on the scale. You might also strive for wellness and the many other benefits associated with Veganism and Fasting. Once you experience it, losing weight becomes merely a consequence of leading a healthier lifestyle.

References

Natalucci G, Riedl S, Gleiss A, Zidek T, Frisch H. Spontaneous 24-h ghrelin secretion pattern in fasting subjects: maintenance of a meal-related pattern. Eur J Endocrinol. 2005;152(6):845-850. doi:10.1530/eje.1.01919

Espelund U, Hansen TK, Højlund K, Beck-Nielsen H, Clausen JT, Hansen BS, Orskov H, Jørgensen JO, Frystyk J. Fasting unmasks a strong inverse association between ghrelin and cortisol in serum: studies in obese and normal-weight subjects. J Clin Endocrinol Metab. 2005 Feb;90(2):741-6. doi: 10.1210/jc.2004-0604. Epub 2004 Nov 2. PMID: 15522942.

Arnason TG, Bowen MW, Mansell KD. Effects of intermittent fasting on health markers in those with type 2 diabetes: A pilot study. World J Diabetes. 2017;8(4):154-164. doi:10.4239/wjd.v8.i4.154

Le LT, Sabaté J. Beyond meatless, the health effects of vegan diets: findings from the Adventist cohorts.

Nutrients. 2014;6(6):2131-2147. Published 2014 May 27. doi:10.3390/nu6062131

Macknin M, Kong T, Weier A, et al. Plant-based, no-added-fat or American Heart Association diets: impact on cardiovascular risk in obese children with hypercholesterolemia and their parents. J Pediatr. 2015;166(4):953-9.e93. doi:10.1016/j.jpeds.2014.12.058

Marosi K, Moehl K, Navas-Enamorado I, et al. Metabolic and molecular framework for the enhancement of endurance by intermittent food deprivation. FASEB J. 2018;32(7):3844-3858. doi:10.1096/fj.201701378RR

Li L, Wang Z, Zuo Z. Chronic intermittent fasting improves cognitive functions and brain structures in mice. PLoS One. 2013;8(6):e66069. Published 2013 Jun 3. doi:10.1371/journal.pone.0066069

Printed in Great Britain
by Amazon